Raising

Raising Hell!!!

Tortured By Mental Illness....!

By Pearl Lilly

Raising Hell!!!

Raising Hell!!!

Tortured By Mental Illness....!

Pearl Lilly

www.pearllilly.com

Raising Hell!!!

Raising Hell!!!

Chapters……..

Ch. 1: Mental Illness.

Ch. 2: In the beginning.

Ch. 3: Changes.

Ch. 4: Call from School.

Ch. 5: Running Away.

Ch. 6: Therapy.

Ch. 7: Mental Illness robbed us!

Ch. 8: Identifying a Body.

Ch. 9: Placement.

Ch. 10: Home.

Ch. 11: Raising Hell All Over Again!!!

Raising Hell!!!

Raising Hell!!!

Pearl Lilly

Little Rock, Arkansas. 72211

pearllilly06@yahoo.com

501-580-9773

All right reserved. No part of this book may be reproduced in any form or by any means what so ever.

10 9 8 7 6 5 4 3 2 1

Copyright©2015 Pearl Lilly

All rights reserved…

pearllilly06@yahoo.com

ISBN-13: 978-1484930175

Raising Hell!!!

Raising Hell!!!

Acknowledgments

I thank my God for giving me the strength to believe within myself and never giving up.

Thanks to my family and friends…I thank you and love you for your continuous support and prayers!

To my readers; thanks for your support for believing in me…

Love you all!!

Pearl Lilly

www.pearllilly.com

Raising Hell!!!

Raising Hell!!!

PROLOGUE

This book is about the struggles of dealing with Mental Illness that my family, friends, and I had endured for so long. Not fully being aware of what mental illness was until being faced with it within my own home.

Having a child suffering from mental illness was painful, because having this beautiful, talented child, who could play a music piece by only hearing it once. One who led her

Raising Hell!!!

Basketball team to victory with her famous 3-points shot.

Raising Hell!!!

Mental Illness can affect anyone, but allowing family, friends, therapist, and physician to help you through it, you're not alone!

Raising Hell!!!

Raising Hell!!!

For My daughter.......

Mental illness robbed you for so long and from your past, but don't allow it to continue to rob you from your future and all of the possibilities!!!!!

I LOVE YOU.......

Raising Hell!!!

Chapter 1

Mental Illness

Mental illness is a difficult thing to understand and that when going through situation when a family member is having mood changes and behaving differently, when tend to think that "Oh, they're just acting out"! When in fact, they may not fully understand what is going on with them.

A lot of families are not prepared to cope with the fact that their loved one is dealing with mental

Raising Hell!!!

illness. Mental illness can be both physically and emotionally draining, causing them to feel "vulnerable" that others may talk about them or even dislike them.

When we think about the fact of mental illness, I think that there are a lot of different stigma that occur within the African American family because, it like when we are having a difficult time, a lot of peoples think that it's because that individual is stupid, crazy, or even just seeking attention from others.

I myself have to say that that is not the case, because dealing with mental illness such as depression,

Raising Hell!!!

causes me to feel bad about the things that had gone through within my life, but it's how I, myself as well as others deal with the depression..

Mental illness can range from that of mild to server form of the disorder. Their symptom can cause the person to have a hard time dealing with things within their life and that sometimes they are able to handle it so they may result to terrible things such as drugs, alcohol, abuse, rage, and even suicide, because they cannot handle their symptoms.

When looking at mental illness, it can range from "depression, bipolar disorder, dementia, schizophrenia and

Raising Hell!!!

anxiety disorders" according to the Department of Medical health, 2015.

Some of the Symptoms causes some changes in people's feelings, thoughts, actions, behaviors, mood disorder and even change their personality.

The person's personal habits will sometimes change causing to sleep a lot or not at all, may even stop eating or eat more than normal. Sometimes they may even stop hanging around peoples and withdrawal from their world.

Raising Hell!!!

Raising Hell!!!

Mental Illness is not the end of the World!!!

Raising Hell!!!

Chapter 2

In The Beginning

In the beginning, things were great and that I couldn't imagine life any better for me and my six children. I had my own home, vehicle, bank account, and a great job.

I thought that despite the fact that I had isolated myself from certain family members that I would still be ok.

There were a lot of reasons that I needed to isolate myself from some family members because, I knew what

Raising Hell!!!

I had gone through, and the emotional, sexual abuse that I had endured and did not want my children to suffer any abuse I like had endured most of my life.

I was able to complete school and take care of my 6 children on my own. It was safe that and dealing with all of the B.S. that I had dealt with, being a single mother was ok.

In the beginning my daughter was a strong healthy kid, who was really loved and cared about. She was the best student and children that a mother would love to have. She was really quite and just an overall beautiful child.

Raising Hell!!!

I think it was around the 7th grade, she was maybe 14 years old when things changed. I never would have thought that I would get a call from the schools' counselor, notifying me that my daughter had missed a total of fifteen days of school and that I needed to come in for an conference with her, teachers, and principal.

My first initial thought was, they had my child confused with another student. But when I arrived at the school and looking at a video on the school's security camera; there she was, skipping with several other students, as well as a fight that she was in with another student.

Raising Hell!!!

I recall how agree I had become, because that really made me more embarrassed that anything. One thing that I had learn was, never to say what your child will and will not do!

After that meeting, I went home to look for my daughter to see what the hell was going on. By the time I got home, who would be home in the living room with a boy.

"Did you lose your God Damn Mind"!!!

We went back and forth, I had forgotten all about her ass skipping and fighting at school.

Raising Hell!!!

I was trying get an understanding of how in the hell, did this child think that she could bring some nigga up in my house and be all laying up like they were married and stuff.

I remember grabbing her, telling her that "I would knock the hell out of you" for disrespecting me.

"Really"!!

I was to through and blown the hell away.

Dealing with her and that young man would take a terrible toll on the family and that I would have never imagine that my child would

Raising Hell!!!

once the sweetest young girl that everyone loved to that of a monster. Life was forever change and now I'm

Raising **H**ell!!!!

Raising Hell!!!

Chapter 3

Changes

There were a lot of changes that the family had gone through. Her behavior at school had went changed from good to bad, behavior at home was not good, as well as the once disrespectful young girl, was now a terror from hell.

My family was having a difficult time dealing with all of the changes that my daughter was putting us through and that it would have only gotten worse. There were times when

Raising Hell!!!

my daughter would start picking with the two younger siblings by punching them, hitting, cursing them, and the constant threats against them as well as on me at times.

    The changes were unbearable; not understanding what in the world was really going on with my child. I just asked God to give us the strength to help us all to get through those changes. I didn't understand why she was doing all of those crazy things during that time.

The changes had manifested within her behaviors from wanting to kill herself and others, to even running away to the point that we did not

Raising Hell!!!

know where she was for days at a time.

I knew that I needed to get help for her. That everything that I was helping her with, talking to her was like it was going out of one ear through the other and nothing seem to have made any difference within her behavior. The changes grew worse than ever before!

She had started to runaway more and more.

She had started talking out her head as if she was the devil himself!

She felt and even thought that we all were out to get her!

Raising Hell!!!

When in fact, we weren't, but you see, mental illness made her think and feel that way. It was a nightmare that I thought would never end!

Raising Hell!!!

Chapter 4

Calls from School!

I remember that I would sit and wait for my daughter, so that I could talk to her about the letters that the school had mailed me on a number of occasions, because after having many conversations with my daughter and the consequences regarding all of her skipping and tardiness that she was continuing to do.

It seemed as if she didn't give a damn if the school and the district

Raising Hell!!!

were mailing me these letters regarding the possibility of me going to jail or even paying multiple fees for her not going to school.

All I ever wanted was for all of my children to go to school and get the best education, which was free and the sad part about it was the fact that school I work for the school district.

I think it didn't matter to my daughter as long as she was able to hang with those no good for nothing friends that continued to get in trouble and some even went in and out of the juvenile system and foster care.

Raising Hell!!!

The calls continued and became piss!

I remembered that I kept calling the school to see what if anything that they could do and if so, "Do it!"

Speaking with the school counselor, she asked that my daughter be picked up and taken to juvenile. At first, I was like No!

It wasn't like she was doing crazy stuff like that and like the other students that she was hanging with.

I just remember that I was so fade up with all of the stuff that she was doing and that I had enough of it

Raising Hell!!!

and the school calling me on a regular basis.

I knew that I needed to make some drastic changes in the way that I was allowing her to continue to skip school and then walk in my house as if she was there all day and every day.

When I approached my daughter about the skipping, her and I had gotten into a verbal altercation, which then lead into a physical one.

I just remember that I grabbed her and slammed her down on the floor to help calm her tail down. Then as soon as I looked away, that child took her fist and wacked me dead on

Raising Hell!!!

the right side of my head. I thought that I had turned into a monster, because all I remember was that I wanted to physically harm that child.

For her to have put her hands on me, I just remember what the elderly peoples had stated many times before.

"Raise your hands up at an adult, you will find yourself pushing up daisies!"

I remember calling one of the other children, asking them to hurry up and call 911, before I murdered my child, because of the way that she was behaving was as if she was some type

Raising Hell!!!

of burglar whom had broken into my home to violently assault me.

When the police had arrived, they had taken her into custody so that they could take her to the hospital to make sure that she wasn't going to harm herself or someone else.

They had asked if she was on some type of drugs or something, because of the way that she was behaving.

I couldn't really answer that because; I myself wondered the same thing. I just remember that I couldn't understand why my child would try to

Raising Hell!!!

attack me, furthermore the more, try to kill me!

In my mind, I felt that this boy that she was going crazy over had given her something or had told her the sweetest shit that she was going absolutely crazy for him and that no matter what his ass said; I was not going to lose my child for his grown dysfunctional ass.

I remember that my daughter was placed in several different types of programs and that all we wanted was for the daughter and sister that we love and known; would come back to us.

Raising Hell!!!

She returned home after a few weeks of treatment and being able to talk with someone that had listened to her regarding everything that she had gone through with being arrested by the police officers and taken away from her family because of her violence and rage toward the officers.

Raising Hell!!!

Chapter 5

Running Away

There were always times that I used to sit ad worry about my daughter. Not know where she was and who she was with. There were many days that I had sat up waiting for my daughter to come home, not realizing that it would be three to five days, and then it was weeks.

I was afraid that my teenage daughter was out there, somewhere and I had nowhere to start looking for her. Running away, was like walking

Raising Hell!!!

to school every day, not realizing that the family would be worried sick about her. I think that the mental illness that she suffers from makes her think and felt that we didn't care or even love her.

Somewhere deep within, my daughter would just disappear and my heart would **STOP!!!**

Why, I used to ask myself that on a regular basis? Asking God, Why was he doing this to her, Doing this to us!!

All my life, I felt that no matter what, I would keep my children safe

Raising Hell!!!

from harm, but how do I keep her safe from herself?

Many days, I recall sitting at the dining room table, thinking that she would be home soon, but she didn't and that made the rage inside of me fell hatred towards her and others that were making her to behave that way.

I wanted to kill them!

I wanted to rip their damn eyes balls out and throw them to the dogs.

Why Me Lord? Why Me?

I remember the empty feeling that I had every time she would leave and not knowing if one day, I would

Raising Hell!!!

have to go and identify a body. I called the police serval times. Of course I had to follow the protocol of waiting 48 hours before they could even take the initial missing person report.

Lord knows, my mind was outer space. Like, I wasn't thinking like that of a normal person.

I recall many days and nights that I had gotten in my car and drove around for hours, some days 5 hours at a time to find my daughter.

I realize now, that I was losing my mind, because I can't even remember half of the place that even

Raising Hell!!!

looked for her. I was just driving and driving hoping and praying to God that I would run into some of her friends and even her. I wouldn't be mad, just happy to see her!

That didn't happen, no time soon. It was probably somewhere like 2 week or so before the police would have located my daughter safe and sound.

There were many other times that she had placed worries upon her family regarding her many escapades of disappearing without a trace.

Many peoples told me, that my child was going to put me in an early

Raising Hell!!!

grave, worrying about her where she was and things like that.

I just cried, because I felt this emptiness of love that was there for my daughter, it ended up becoming anger and bitterness towards her.

As I am sitting here thinking, I could never understand why my daughter felt the need to have run away from home.

I thought that she was doing such a wonderful job in school, because she was getting straight A's in her grades, was on the school's basketball team and of course a great 3 point shooter, as well as having the

Raising Hell!!!

ability that God had given her to play the keyboard by ear. Meaning, that she was able to listen to a piece and then turn around and play that same song.

I learned that there were many reasons that teenagers would think about running away, but I just didn't understand why my daughter felt that her home wasn't safe enough for her.

Running away from home was as if she was not a member of our family and her disappearance became routine.

It became serious when, one day late December, I went to the

Raising Hell!!!

grocery store. Upon my arrival, I looked in the children's bedroom to make sure that they were ok. When I looked in my daughter's room, she was gone.

So, I looked around the house, but there were no signs of her. Her coat was still in her bedroom. Her shoes where in front of the front door, and everything was in place.

BUT WHERE WAS MY DAUGHTER??

I panic, due to the fact that it was only 16° outside, with snow everywhere and my daughter did not

Raising Hell!!!

have anything on. Not even a freaking coat or clothing!

She was missing at that time for about 3 weeks or so.

The fear of the unknown had taken over my body and robbed my mind!

That was when I knew it was time to get **<u>HELP</u>**!!!!!!!!!!!!!!!!!!!!

Raising Hell!!!

Raising Hell!!!

GOD, PLACE YOUR HAND UPON MY DAUGHTER, SO THA THE PAIN WITHIN HER HEART CAN BE LET FREE!!!

Raising Hell!!!

Chapter 6

Therapy

I knew that I needed to get my daughter the help that she so much needed as well as for the rest of the family. I remember coming up, that African-American don't go to NO therapist and talk about what was or is going on within the family. You just don't do that!

So, for a long all of the shit that we were going through, I just kept inside and within the home. Mostly due to the fact that I was

Raising Hell!!!

SOOOOO damn embarrassed, that I we were going through all of that shit!

It was like every chance that my daughter started to act like a fool, and **RAISING HELL**, she knew that I would get in my feelings and just shut myself off from the world!

Things had gotten worse, I knew that no matter what peoples had thought about me and my children that I need to get help and I did. Yes, we were laughed at and looked at as if we were really crazy, more so my children, because they were a part of me!

That in it self made peoples think that we were crazy. I guess, I didn't care,

Raising Hell!!!

as long as we got the help that we needed!

Raising Hell!!!

Chapter 7

Mental Illness robbed us!

It was a quite Saturday afternoon, the house was a rest, all of the children were outside enjoying a bright clear grey sky as they played, running around like young brown squirrel searching for freedom. I sat, with my back against the pavement of the wall, as I watched them run free as if they had no care in the world.

As the shadow from the light peaking in the room; binding by the limited space due the clothing and

Raising Hell!!!

black plastic bags, that belong to my middle sister in need of a place to crest her body.

Not sure why my mother would allow her space to be invaded by my sister, like a thief stealing from a corner store.

I always wanted to tell my mother how I felt as well as the other siblings, but in the respect to our mother, as to that of the Pope, himself, obedience is a must. I try to maintain my feelings of rage, like a burning fire that can destroy a family's sanctuary.

Raising Hell!!!

My daughter, tells me like the others, of course in anger and rage, "I'll Kill You", in reaction of not getting what she wants.

I try not to reveal my frustration towards my daughter while my daughter devours my love and kindness like a snake swallowing his prey; consumes my soul like an innocence mouse as it travels through the wooded fields in search for safety.

I try to stay to myself and not express the way that I am feeling, because I know in my heart that my daughter is only out to destroy our family and the rest of us like the terrors that plague on this country.

Raising Hell!!!

My daughter, which I don't understand and nothing like the rest of my children, brought up the same manner, but her demeanor of that cold-hearted killer, just returns to our lives to torture us and keeps an hold me like an inmate in a jail cell.

My daughter, who suffers from mental illness, keeps us all as her prisoners within her head, the feelings of anger towards her because it robbed us of the good time.

Ten years ago, very intelligent young lady, who could play music by sound, humming bird buzzing beautifully; sounds of ocean calling for peace.

Raising Hell!!!

My daughter, I missed dearly is kidnapped by mental illness!

I tried my best to help her as well as other peoples who believed in her. Even still today, as I put my life on hold to care for her two helpless little sons, but how do I express the hatred towards the monster that lives within her, who continues to hunt us like prey!

I am angry that our life was turned upside down like a damn tornado before us. Many beautiful days were destroyed from the destruction of her path that my daughter had created.

Raising Hell!!!

Nothing was standing tall anymore; we all seem to have gotten knocked down like a bull dozer knocking down an abandon building.

We have all became lifeless like the weeping willow that steams from the bark of the tree, floating in the storm of the unknown twister before us; and I don't mean to sound bad, but being torture by the demon that lives inside of my daughter for so long that she is no more human.

I look at my daughter as if, something in her head would tell me that she coming home, for that moment of peace, I validate her presence.

Raising Hell!!!

Quite like a mouse, tall as a tree, until that voice within her mind tells her that we, especially I, don't love her; then it brings out the monster that has the voice of demons throughout the day like at night that can wake up the dead. I don't think my daughter realizes the hurt her siblings and I are feeling.

As I am filled with hope, that one day my daughter will leave the darkness within her mind and return to the light of day; where we all are happy and free.

I wish that I didn't feel the way that I do, but it is hard when we are living with terror!

Raising Hell!!!

If I knew how to have a better understanding of why I find the need to always rescue her, but while we all are drowning, while she continues to destroy us, then maybe, I could feel better, think better, and have a better thinking process for her instead of hatred!

My daughter, victim of mental illness, empowered by super hero strength when in rage, bringing on the fears that stops us in our tracks, because of the unknown contact we will have with her.

One assault was so bad, blood flowing from my head like a river.

Raising Hell!!!

In the mist of the terror, body features change, facial express scary like a horror monster with demon eyes, strength like a bear, clawing me until I pushed her off of me.

I still don't understand this mental illness as it robs her mind and soul, but I try to forgive her until the next time the demons awaken inside of her!

I never realize the fear of my daughters' mental illness until late March 2007, when she was missing for a little over a month. Not realizing if she was dead or alive, was one of many fears that I endured along with

Raising Hell!!!

the other children that cared and love her.

Raising Hell!!!

Mental Illness……..

Living with mental illness, is like living life with having no lights on inside and when the illness is on, everything within is dark.

Living in a world full of darkness or realizing the terror that is lurking to come out. Not even knowing what will transpire! Mental illness robbed us like a robber in the night.

Raising Hell!!!

Chapter 8

Identifying a Body

I worries of my daughters' where about had taken a toll of me. I found myself going to see my therapist on a regular basis. Sometime two or three times a week. I realize now that worrying only was making me ill myself.

I knew that I had to allow the police and everyone else to do their jobs and going on living as if my daughters was away at a week-long camping trip. But that in itself was very hard to tackle. I went to work,

Raising Hell!!!

complete my college courses of course with a low grade of "D". I had to admit to myself, that nothing matter, not even life at that point.

But I knew that I had to keep moving forward. I would sit in my bedroom, along the side of my bed and cry. I was so angry at her, at god, and even t myself.

I knew that I had done this best that I could have done with her, like with the other children before and after her. Treat them all the same!

It was late, I had just put the other children down for bed; then lay down on the sofa, for a little while.

Raising Hell!!!

Just to lay there, to allow my brain and soul to just lay there and rest, rest for just one moment without thinking about anything.

As I crest the pillow of the sofa, I allowed my body to sink into the sofa, and rest.

I remember it feeling so good to just lay there and not have a worry for just that one moment. I heard my heart beating in every beat.

The joyful sounds of crickets as they jumped through the night.

Resting my and rest!

Suddenly, there was a loud knock on my front door and all I could think

Raising Hell!!!

of, that it was my daughter coming home. It didn't matter where she was or had been; just having her home was all that had matter to me.

I would ask no question at all!

I remember rushing to the front door, as I reached it and turn the nob; I notice a tall figure standing there before me through the peak hole.

Suddenly, my heart dropped!

I open the door and there standing, the LPD officer, with his face hanging low. A squeaky voice came out saying "Mrs. Lilly". I responded, "Yes, That's me.'

Raising Hell!!!

He asked if I could come with him. I wasn't sure and I didn't know nor like the police at that time. It was mostly fear within me that kept my feet stuck to the floor.

The police officer asked me if I was alright and I told him that I was ok….that I was afraid to go. I knew in my heart that I couldn't go alone. So I called some family and friends to go with me to the hospital and then to a home located on Barns Rd.

Upon my arrival at the hospital, I knew that I was not prepare to see this body and to think that It could have been the body of my daughter, my baby.

Raising Hell!!!

Every step that I had taken was like eternity!

My heart was beating as if it was jumping out of my body.

The nurse had called my name and I knew that I couldn't do it, but I took those steps as if I was taking a journey and when I reached the room, I dropped to my knees and asked God, to please help me.

Don't let that individual that was no more, be my child Lord.

I asked the nurse to describe her hair, and if she had sharp teeth like that of a vampire.

The nurse replied, NO!!

Raising Hell!!!

Then I knew that wasn't my daughter. She was the only child of mines with those unique features.

I sign with relief that it wasn't my child. I got up and walked towards my family and friends.

We left the hospital to head to Barns Rd.

When we arrived, there were others families that were there and somewhere crying.

I didn't know what to think about what was going on. All could think have been that I hope whoever was upstairs in that house, was not my daughter.

Raising Hell!!!

It wasn't and I continued to pray for my family and myself as well as for the other families that were there.

I felt as if my life ad past right by my eye. Lord I thank you for that not being my child.

Chapter 9

Placement

When my daughter eventually returned home, I just hug her and that I didn't fuse at her or anything. I just told her that I'll get the help that she needed and that everything was going to be ok.

I went to talk with her therapist and the Ingham County Community Children Mental Health located there on South Cedar Street in Lansing, Michigan. I receive the help that she

Raising Hell!!!

need from awesome therapy's and other support services that were put in place for us.

The team was all wonderful; I wish that I could say their name, because they all provided services from counseling to placement.

They even attended court session and provided the children with fun activities and support group therapies and Project Clay activities and memberships.

My daughter was place in serval settings and that my daughter was given all of the help that she needed. I want to say thank you to the

Raising Hell!!!

following individuals for assisting my family: Linda M, Cristy B, Nancy, and Shalonda. Dagmar, Ingham County Children Health Services, and others.

Raising Hell!!!

Friends are those who don't cast judgement, they offer support and wisdom.

Raising Hell!!!

Chapter 10
Home

My daughter was allowed to come home for visit and then go back before a certain time and then that lasted for several months.

As the months past, there were many ongoing episodes that the family had gone through with my daughter. There were assaults and stealing and running away started up again. I didn't understand why?

Raising Hell!!!

Home should be a place of peace and happiness, but for my daughter, she felt that there were things that kept here running and angry.

In her mind, she felt hat the family was out to get her and that even though raising her the same way as the other children, her mind played her against us.

You see, with mental illness, it robbed her mind, making her think that we were demons out to destroy her.

To help save my daughter, I continued to reach out to her and get

Raising Hell!!!

the services that she needed and also for the rest of us.

There still were situation that caused for my daughter to feel like she needed to run away, which resulted with the Lansing Police Department to have get involved.

The home that we once had was no more; I lost my home t that I worked so hard to have for my children. Because of the behavior of my daughter, we were face with her going to jail for 6 years or was asked to live the state of Michigan. I knew that I was tired of Michigan, so I quit my job, moved my

Raising Hell!!!

family and never looked back. The home that we had, was no more!

We moved to Greenwood, Mississippi, and started a new life there until the monsters within my daughter awaken again. Living life the same way as we had in Lansing, Michigan…..was an nightmare.

Raising Hell!!!

Raising Hell!!!

From Michigan to Mississippi to Arkansas and now Georgia!!!

Will the monster ever go away?

Raising Hell!!!

Chapter 11

Raising Hell All Over Again!!!

The nightmare never seems to be destroyed. We were hunted by its presence every time that my daughter was around. Yes, there were many days that she was ok and we never had to deal with the mental illness that robbed her mind.

Until one day, she felt that we were all talking about her and some triggered that demon within.

It was awake and all hell broke out. Telling her brother on a daily basis

Raising Hell!!!

that she will kill him and for him to watch his back was like a routine.

The names that she had given me of

BITCH THIS…

BITCH THAT…

MOTHER FUCKER THAT and THIS…

The monster was out…yelling and screaming at me.

Then one day…the attacked her sister while holding her niece….fighting match broke out and police was called…

Raising Hell!!!

The DEMON was out….

Out to destroy everything that I had worked so hard to burry.

Demon cast its claws on my child…

The innocence daughter that tried to help me save, was frighten by the glowing of the police gun…He was going to shot my oldest daughter, because the monster in my middle daughter wanted her dead.

I can't save my daughter from the demon because of the destruction of the others. I have to let you go, in order to save us!!!!

Raising Hell!!!

I WILL ALWAYS LOVE YOU, but you have to love yourself and receive the help that you need.

I will always be here for you…..

Raising Hell All Over Again!!!

Raising Hell!!!

Raising Hell!!!

<u>Notes</u>

Raising Hell!!!

<u>Notes</u>

Raising Hell!!!

<u>**Notes**</u>

Raising Hell!!!

<u>Notes</u>

Raising Hell!!!

<u>Notes</u>

Raising Hell!!!

<u>Notes</u>

Raising Hell!!!

Raising Hell!!!

PEACE!!!!!!

Raising Hell!!!

Raising Hell!!!

By Pearl Lilly

Raising Hell!!!

Raising Hell!!!

Raising Hell!!!

<u>Notes</u>

Raising Hell!!!

<u>Notes</u>

By Pearl Lilly

Raising Hell!!!

Raising Hell!!!

Also By Pearl Lilly

Lost Soul of A Child

God, Give Me Strength

Surviving It All!!

Raising Hell

Raising Hell!!!

Raising Hell!!!

Raising Hell!!!

Also By Pearl Lilly

Lost Soul of A Child

God, Give Me Strength

Surviving It All!!

Raising Hell

Raising Hell!!!

Raising Hell!!!

Raising Hell!!!

Made in the USA
Columbia, SC
04 June 2025